Table of Contents

The earliest recorded reference to respiratory distress – a disorder characterized by "noisy breathing" (wheezing?) is found in China in 2600 BC.

The Babylonian "Code of Hammurabi" recorded symptoms of breathlessness: "If a man's lungs pant with his work." (1792-1750 BC).

Hippocrates (~400 BC) was the first to use the term "Asthma" (Greek for "wind" or "to blow") for panting and respiratory distress. He is considered to be the physician who identified the relationship between the environment and respiratory disease correlating climate and location with illness. Some suggest he was the first allergist.

When Alexander the Great invaded India, smoking the herb stramonium (an anticholinergic agent related to ipratropium and tiotropium currently used in inhalers) was used to relax the lungs.

Roman doctors described asthma as gasping and the inability to breathe without making noise. They noted "if from running or any other work, the breath becomes difficult, it is called asthma." Pliny the elder (~ 50 AD) observed that pollen was a source of respiratory difficulty and recommended the use of "ephedra" (forerunner of ephedrine) in red wine as an asthma remedy. Unfortunately, he also suggested that drinking the blood of wild horses and eating 21 millipedes soaked in honey could help.

The Jewish Talmud (200-500 AD) counseled "drinking three weights of hiltith," a resin of the carrot family as a therapy for asthma. Maimonides (1135-1204 AD), Jewish scholar and Saladin's physician treated the Egyptian's son for asthma. His "Treatise on Asthma" prescribed rest, good personal hygiene and environment, avoidance of opium, a small quantity of wine and a special diet. Nuts, fruit, milk, cool vegetables and legumes (peanuts are a member of this family) were forbidden, while "The soup of fat hens" was considered beneficial.

Tobacco introduced from the America's to Europe (1500's), was used to induce coughing and expectorate mucus. In Central America, Aztecs ingested an ephedra containing plant to clear mucus and, in South America, Incas treated asthma with a cocaine-like dried leaf. In the 1800's, Arsenic was prescribed for respiratory conditions. In the early 1900's, allergy immunotherapy was first introduced to treat asthma.

Asthma medicines of the 1940's and 1950's consisted of epinephrine injections (adrenaline) and aminophylline tablets or suppositories. In the 1960's oral combinations were the staples of chronic therapy. Inhalation of epinephrine (Primatene) and isoproterenol (Isuprel) were used as rescue agents. Oral prednisone was and continues to be prescribed for severe disease.

Since the Allergy and Asthma Medical Group & Research Center was founded in 1969, many therapeutic advances have occurred. Inhaled bronchodilator medications are less likely to stimulate the heart and are available in both short and long acting formulations. Inhaled corticosteroids target the underlying inflammation and minimize the potential cortisone side effects seen with the tablet and liquid products. Our clinical research department is currently actively evaluating new asthma therapies that promise to further benefit patients.

According to the American College of Allergy, Asthma, and Immunology, an estimated 26 million people in America suffer from asthma, including seven million children. This makes asthma the leading chronic disease in children. Consequently, asthma causes a staggering average of 13.8 million school absences per year. For adults, the annual economic loss in work productivity is estimated at $81.9 billion.

Symptoms can be triggered by allergens and non-allergens. Allergic triggers can include outdoor allergens such as pollen, grass, and trees, or indoor allergens like dust and pet dander. Non-allergic triggers consist of weather, exercise, illness, stress, physical displays of emotion that affect normal breathing (e.g. shouting, screaming, laughing), and environmental irritants such as smoke, pollutants, and chemicals.

Other triggers include illnesses which affect the respiratory system like the common cold, drugs and over-the-counter medications such as aspirin and ibuprofen, or food additives like preservatives (however, food triggers are rare).

Asthma is often confused as an allergy since the symptoms are only seen when triggered. However, asthma is a chronic disease and is always present even when a patient is not experiencing symptoms. Thus, allergens may trigger symptoms but are not the cause of asthma.

Unfortunately, there is no known cause of asthma. Genetic abnormalities are considered the most likely culprit.

Anyone can develop asthma, yet some people are more susceptible and may experience more severe symptoms. For example, the disease is more common in children than adults, yet adults are four times more likely to die from it. In addition, boys are more likely to get asthma than girls, but women are more likely than men.

Puerto Ricans and African-Americans are at the highest risk of developing the disease, being hospitalized, and dying from it, often due to poor environmental conditions. Around 3,300 Americans die from asthma each year.

Asthma is a chronic inflammatory disease in the lungs, characterized by restricted breathing. The most common symptoms include coughing, wheezing, shortness of breath, chest tightness, and difficulty breathing. Depending on the frequency of these symptoms and how severely they degrade quality of life, patients can also experience depression.

Asthma is a complex disease affecting the lungs that can be managed but cannot be cured.1 Asthma can be controlled well in most people most of the time, although some people may have more persistent problems. Asthma attacks (exacerbations) occur when symptoms worsen, and those affected can require hospitalisation. 1 There are different types of asthma; more than half of patients have Type 2 asthma, an important distinction because the causes of inflammation that result in Type 2 asthma symptoms have been clearly identified. Epidemiology There are 334 million people with asthma across the globe today, The number of asthma patients could grow by a third within ten years due to better diagnosis and changes in diet, housing, pollution and exposure to nature. A quarter of a million people die from asthma each year worldwide, or one person every two minutes. 5,7 The annual costs of healthcare and lost productivity on account of asthma are €33.9 billion in the EU. Of this, direct costs for drugs, inpatient and outpatient care were €19.5 billion, and indirect costs €14.4 billion. A small fraction of people with asthma are estimated to have severe disease15,18 yet they absorb over 50% of the treatments costs15,16 and account for nearly 40% of asthma deaths. 17 It is estimated that 10% of asthma patients have severe disease that is not controlled by medication. Costs for uncontrolled patients can be more than double those for controlled patients.14 Causes of asthma and triggers Asthma results from inflammation of the bronchioli (which carry air in and out of the lungs), leading to restricted airflow.1 In asthma patients, the inflamed bronchioli are more sensitive to particles in the air. When an asthma attack occurs, mucus production is increased, muscles of the bronchioli become tight and the lining of the air passages swells, reducing airflow and producing the characteristic wheezing sound associated with asthma.

CAUSES OF ASTHMA

Although research has revealed much about asthma over recent decades, we still don't really understand what causes the disease. We have more and more pieces of intriguing information about asthma, but we don't know how those pieces will end up fitting together. Some pieces will be causes; some will be contributing factors; and some will be dead ends.

UI Health's asthma clinic is proud to participate in the ongoing research that will someday help us fully understand the factors that lead to this disease.

Through ongoing research, we continue to draw closer to the day when all the pieces are in place. When we know what causes asthma, we will be much better equipped to prevent it and possibly to cure it.

Until then, we have some interesting puzzle pieces to work with.

Genetics

One risk factor for asthma is a condition called atopy, which is essentially a predisposition to be allergic to things. The evidence is quite clear that heredity is partially responsible for a person having atopy.

We know that genes contribute to atopy, which is a risk factor for asthma. But are there specific asthma genes?

The answer is but the evidence is convincing that asthma is not a "single-gene" disease. Involvement of several different genes, though, in such asthma components as airway hyperresponsiveness and non-atopy-related inflammation seems likely but has not been proven.

A large percentage — probably about one-third — of babies and young children will experience wheezing at some point, usually during a viral respiratory infection. Some but not all of these children go on to have chronic asthma. It is unclear just what the role of the viral infection is, but it is possible that it is part of the cause of asthma.

The viruses that most commonly cause wheezing in infants are RSV (respiratory syncytial virus) and parainfluenza virus. In slightly older children, rhinovirus — the virus responsible for the common cold — is a frequent cause of wheezing.

Air Quality

The evidence is clear that air pollution can have a negative effect on the breathing of people who already have asthma.

Particulate matter (tiny particles of liquids and solids) in the air has also been shown to have adverse effects on breathing in general, particularly (but not exclusively) in people who already have respiratory problems.

It is unfortunately very difficult, though, to do research that can tell us whether or not air pollution actually causes asthma in people who don't already have the disease.

Cigarette Smoke

The case against cigarette smoke is even stronger than the case against air pollution.

It is thought that exposure to cigarette smoke in childhood contributes both directly and indirectly to the development of asthma.

In study after study, children exposed to tobacco smoke in the home have been shown to have higher rates of hospitalizations for respiratory illness. Serious respiratory illness before the age of 2 is an important risk factor for asthma.

It is believed that cigarette smoke also has a more direct role in causing asthma, either through effects on the immune system, on the formation of the airways, or both. Exposure to cigarette smoke in utero (through the mother smoking during pregnancy) appears to be at least as harmful as exposure in the home during infancy and early childhood. The risks also rise as the amount of cigarette smoke exposure rises due to an effect called "dose response" (usually seen as evidence of a causal link).

First World/Third World Difference

Another observation that may hold clues to the causes of asthma is that asthma is much more common in industrialized nations — such as the United States — than in the developing world. We still do not know why this is so. It is unlikely to be related to the genetic makeup of the populations, since descendants of immigrants from developing nations to industrialized ones have similar asthma rates to those in their adoptive country.

Several explanations have been suggested to explain the higher prevalence of asthma in industrialized nations:

• Higher rates of different infectious diseases in the developing world — from measles to malaria, bacteria to parasitic worms — may somehow affect people's immune systems in a way that is protective against asthma.

• Spending more time indoors than their developing nation counterparts may expose children in industrialized nations to allergens or pollutants that contribute to asthma.

• Excess body weight may be a risk factor for asthma. And children in developing nations are thinner than children in industrialized nations.

How Might Causes of Asthma Fit Together?

One theory for explaining how asthma is caused involves a combination of underlying susceptibility with environmental exposures, often referred to as "hits." Under such a model, it is believed that a person who is not born with a genetic susceptibility to asthma will never get the disease, no matter what the environment. A person who is born genetically vulnerable to asthma also may escape the disease if he or she is not exposed to enough "hits" in the environment to bring it out. Asthma occurs, by this theory, only when a person both is susceptible (through heredity) and experiences those factors (still unidentified) that cause the disease to manifest itself.

This is all rather complex, but the picture may in fact be more complicated still. Some scientists believe that what we call "asthma" is actually several different diseases, caused in different ways. It is possible, for instance, that asthma that begins in infancy or childhood could be something else entirely from asthma that comes on in adulthood. Or perhaps asthma in people with allergies could be a different entity from asthma in people who are not allergic. These are some of the questions that asthma researchers are currently attempting to address.

A number of factors can increase the chance of developing asthma, including:

• A family history of asthma or other related allergic conditions, such as food allergy or hay fever

• Having another allergic condition
• Childhood bronchiolitis

• Childhood exposure to tobacco smoke, particularly if exposure occurs during pregnancy

• Being born prematurely, especially if ventilator support was required

• Having a low birth weight as a result of restricted growth within the womb Triggers can be anything that irritates the lungs.

When asthma patients encounter triggers, the airways narrow and the muscles tighten around them. An increase in the production of sticky mucus (phlegm) also occurs. Common triggers include:

• Respiratory tract infections, particularly viral infections affecting the upper airways, such as colds and flu

• Allergens, including pollen, dust mites, animal fur or feathers

- Airborne irritants, including cigarette smoke, chemical fumes and atmospheric pollution

- Medicines, particularly non-steroidal anti-inflammatory drugs (NSAIDs) and beta blockers

- Emotions, including stress or laughing

- Foods containing sulphites, e.g. concentrated fruit juice, jam, prawns and many processed or precooked meals

- Weather conditions, including sudden changes in temperature, cold air and poor air quality

- Indoor conditions, including mould or damp, house dust mites and chemicals in carpets and flooring materials

- Exercise

- Food allergies, including allergies to nuts or other food items

Symptoms and diagnosis

Asthma symptoms can range from mild to moderate or severe. The main symptoms of asthma are wheezing, shortness of breath, a tight chest and coughing. Most people will only experience occasional symptoms, but symptoms are harder to control in those with severe asthma, and they may have problems almost all the time.

There are a number of ways to diagnose asthma, including lung function tests (spirometry, peak expiratory flow test), airway responsiveness, inflammation tests, and allergy tests.

Severe asthma

Severe asthma can be defined as asthma that requires treatment with high dose inhaled corticosteroids (ICS) plus a second controller (and/or systemic corticosteroids) to prevent it from becoming 'uncontrolled' or which remains 'uncontrolled' despite this therapy. Asthma control is ranked by doctors according to lung function, symptoms and the need for reliever medication, as controlled, partly controlled and uncontrolled.

Researchers believe severe asthma is linked to a variety of factors: genetic inheritance, the age of asthma onset, the duration of disease, exacerbations, sinus disease and inflammatory characteristics. Many patients have difficulty breathing most of the time, as well as frequent, life-threatening attacks needing hospital admissions. Severe asthma is a complex, unpredictable disease. Work and social life become limited and every-day activities such as climbing stairs or leaving the house can be a challenge.

Most people with severe asthma are treated with a 'one-size-fits-all' approach, which often doesn't control their daily symptoms or improve outcomes. Patients cycle through different medicines or add on new treatments to find one that relieves their symptoms, but they do not address the root cause. Not only do many patients with severe asthma not respond to conventional treatments, many develop adverse effects from their sustained or repeated use. These adverse events include diabetes, obesity, osteoporosis and depression.

Asthma is a heterogeneous disease. The various forms of asthma result from specific molecular pathways in the immune system and the effects that these have on different types of inflammation in the tissues of the lungs.

Among patients with severe asthma, the majority have Type 2. This category derives its name from increased levels of type 2 inflammatory signals. 19 Type 2 inflammation results from the action of a specific group of molecular messengers (cytokines) produced by the immune system, IL-13, IL-5 and IL-4. An important mediator of Type 2 asthma is IL-13, a protein messenger released by cells that causes inflammation. By targeting the IL-13 pathway, we have the potential to block the development of a wide range of symptoms that are most important to severe asthma patients and that they experience nearly every day. Blocking IL-13 activity has a broad impact on key mechanisms (such as mucus production, airway inflammation, narrowing and hyper-responsiveness) and the day-to-day symptoms. This could include improvement in breathing, relief from daily symptoms, reduced limitations on daily activities, less time spent awake at night, less use of rescue medication and reduced need for medical attention and intervention.

Treatment

Likely patient response to treatment is untested in the majority of cases, so conventional treatment is administered in a stepwise approach, following successive treatment failure. Asthma treatment starts with reliever therapy, followed by the addition of preventer medications, as required. In poorly controlled asthma, other treatments may be added to the patient's medication regimen. Treatment doses are reviewed and altered to achieve the best control using the lowest dose.

Reliever medication is taken via an inhaler to relieve asthma symptoms quickly. Most often, these inhalers contain a short-acting beta agonist (SABA) which works by relaxing the muscles surrounding the narrowed airways.

Preventer inhalers work over time to reduce the amount of inflammation and sensitivity of the airways, and reduce the chances of asthma attacks occurring. They must be used regularly (typically twice or occasionally once daily) and indefinitely to keep asthma under control. Most often, preventer inhalers contain inhaled corticosteroids.

Add-on therapies are introduced if a patient's asthma does not respond to initial treatment. The dose of preventer medication may be increased, or an inhaler containing a long-acting reliever (long-acting bronchodilator/long-acting beta2-agonist, or LABA) may be prescribed.

Additional treatments include leukotriene receptor antagonists, theophyllines, oral steroids and injectable monoclonal antibodies. Bronchial thermoplasty may also be used. Bronchial thermoplasty works by destroying some of the muscles surrounding the airways in the lungs, which can reduce their ability to narrow the airways.

The role of personalised treatment approaches in asthma

Identifying and targeting treatments to specific types of a disease or patient group is called Personalised Healthcare. Already widely applied in cancer treatment, Personalised Healthcare could provide severe asthma patients with the confidence that their medicine is right for them. The way asthma is treated will change dramatically with several new treatments becoming available in the next decade. Treatments are needed that target the critical underlying mechanism responsible for different types of asthma. This in turn may eliminate the cost of trying different medicines to find one that works, and may reduce the side effects and the burden for the patient from the use of multiple therapies to relieve symptoms.

Presence of Type 2 messenger molecules cannot be detected with commercially-available tests, but IL-13 activity produces a protein called periostin that can be detected in the blood as a reliable biomarker for Type 2 asthma. Periostin is the most promising biomarker for Type 2 asthma. By knowing that a patient has Type 2 asthma, physicians could confidently prescribe a Type 2-specific treatment.

Before diving into how CBD may treat asthma, it is important to know how asthma works and is currently treated.

Pathophysiology of Asthma

Asthma is characterized by inflammation in the bronchial tubes, causing difficulty breathing. Inflammation is caused by the presence of immune cells called T-helper cells (Th1 and Th2). These cells produce proinflammatory proteins called cytokines and cytokines are produced when the lungs experience a trigger.

This immune response is abnormal. For healthy individuals, allergens cause no problem. However, when an allergen or other substance enters the lungs of an asthma patient, the immune system perceives the substance as foreign and triggers its inflammatory response.

Another characteristic of asthma is hyperre activity of the airways. In patients with asthma, their airways contract too much and too easily when a trigger is introduced. This action causes wheezing, chest tightness, and other asthmatic symptoms.

Asthma patients also have excess mucus secreted in their lungs, worsening symptoms. Excess mucus is associated with the rising levels of IL-13, a cytokine protein. As this cytokine rises in the lungs, excess mucus is secreted, adding further obstruction to the airways.

Medication for Asthma

No cure is currently available for asthma.

If undiagnosed and not appropriately treated, the disease can lead to death; however, death is often easily avoidable. Several medications exist to manage symptoms. Patients will often have two medications on hand, one for long-term management and another for fast relief of symptoms.

The quick-acting medications are bronchodilators which open up the airways and help remove mucus. Long-term medications are often corticosteroids, such as Symbicort, Flovent, and Advair.

Steroids are powerful drugs and can be dangerous if misused.

If used too long, these medications may cause significant side effects such as infections in the mouth, a weakened immune system increasing the risk of infections, a rise in blood sugar which may lead to diabetes, and stunted growth in children.

Additionally, many patients cannot control or can only partially control their asthma with medication. Especially in cases of severe asthma, patients find little to no relief with medication.

This fact and the potential dangers of prolonged use of medication have created the need to explore and develop novel therapies to more effectively treat asthma.

Fortunately, CBD has positive research behind it that demonstrates it may be a safe and effective way to manage asthma and prevent attacks.

Studies On CBD Treating Asthma

The following studies illustrate the effects of CBD and the endocannabinoid system (the bodily system CBD interacts with) on asthma:

Evaluation of CBD for Asthmatic Inflammation

In the Brazilian university study noted earlier, researchers tested CBD's anti-inflammatory effects on asthma in rats. Twenty-one rats were split into three groups, with one group receiving CBD.

The researchers measured the levels of several cytokines to test CBD's effectiveness.

CBD was found to inhibit the production of all but one cytokine, resulting in significantly decreased inflammation. The cytokines CBD suppressed in the study are also found in human asthma, which encouraged researchers that CBD's anti-inflammatory effect will translate to humans.

The study also noted that past research has shown CBD is well tolerated by humans even when administered chronically, indicating CBD is a potentially safer treatment than medication.

Review of Cannabinoids for Inflammation and Inflammatory Pain

A 2012 study conducted by the University of Florence in Italy explored the role of the endocannabinoid system in asthma.

The research found the activation of cannabinoid receptors on the nerve endings of bronchi acted like a bronchodilator, which opens the airways and allows for unrestricted breathing. It was also concluded that preventing the breakdown of endocannabinoids can reduce pain caused by inflammation.

Since CBD helps activate these receptors, CBD has the potential to be a bronchodilator and an effective analgesic.

Activation of Cannabinoid Receptors in Preventing Asthmatic Reaction

Another study by the University of Florence on guinea pigs aimed to evaluate the role of cannabinoid receptors (CB1 and CB2) in preventing asthmatic symptoms.

The study concluded that both receptors were involved in protecting the lungs and targeting them could be a potential preventative therapy for asthma patients.

A New, Breakthrough Study

As a result of the limited yet promising research above, CIITECH (a biotech company based in the UK and Israel) has funded professors from the Multidisciplinary Center on Cannabinoid Research of the Hebrew University of Jerusalem to conduct their own study.

Asthma expert Dr. Francesca Levi-Schaffer and cannabis researcher Dr. Raphael Mechoulam will be working together to study CBD's potential as a therapy for symptoms of asthma.

The study will test how CBD affects asthma in humans for the first time. The preliminary results of the research should be coming out in the near future.

Israel was one of the first countries to legalize medical marijuana and is one of the world leaders in cannabis research with a government-sponsored cannabis research and development program. As a result, the university has conducted many cannabis studies and is a leader in the field.

Results from this study have the potential to provide significantly more scientific and societal legitimacy to CBD, especially since the study's announcement received considerable media attention. CIITECH is confident the results will be convincing, entitling an article on their website, "We're going to prove cannabis can treat asthma."

Clifton Flack, founder of CIITECH, said he wants to create CBD food supplements based on the research. Creating food supplements instead of medication will save the company time and millions of dollars in regulatory approvals while also providing a product that is widely accessible to consumers.

Professor Levi-Schaffer said an inhaled type of CBD medication could be produced as well.

How CBD Treats Asthma

When choosing a specific CBD product, it is important to go with a reputable brand. Check out our Receptra Naturals review for our take on a trustworthy premium CBD brand.

CBD treats asthma by activating receptors in the endocannabinoid system (the body's natural source for cannabinoids). By activating these receptors, CBD produces its therapeutic effects. CBD's potential effects include the potential to decrease inflammation, inhibit mucus production, reduce airway obstruction, and prevent asthma symptoms.

CBD as an Anti-inflammatory

According to the Brazilian study, CBD has the potential to reduce inflammation in asthma patients. T-helper cells find their way to the respiratory system and produce cytokines when responding to an asthmatic trigger, such as an allergen.

In turn, cytokines produce inflammation which results in shortness of breath and difficulty breathing.

CBD is an anti-inflammatory as it suppresses the responses of T-helper cells. As a result, cytokines are drastically reduced and inflammation subsides, allowing patients to breathe easier. CBD may also reduce the pain associated with inflammation by activating endocannabinoid receptors.

Tumor necrosis factor (TNF) also plays a role in inflammation and adds to the severity of asthma. TNF is another type of cytokine that causes inflammation and influences other cells to do so as well. CBD was found to specifically lower TNF levels and reduce overall inflammation.

CBD Inhibits Mucus Production

Mucus adds to the severity of asthma symptoms and contributes to the obstruction of airways. The introduction of cytokines causes the excess mucus. The cytokine protein IL-13 is widely considered to be the cause of the occurrence.

Fortunately, CBD has been shown to specifically reduce IL-13 levels in the lungs. This effect allows patients to more easily expel mucus from their body via coughing and prevents excess production.

CBD May Prevent Airway Obstruction

The airways in asthma patients tend to be hyperreactive and contract too easily. This often leads to obstructed airways. A study by the Institute for Clinical Pharmacology in Germany showed that an endocannabinoid neurotransmitter called anandamide could restrain this obstruction.

When asthma is induced by a trigger, anandamide increases in a fluid created by the bronchi. The level of anandamide present correlates with the severity of obstruction and inflammation in the airways. For example, if the concentration of anandamide was high, the severity of the obstruction was low.

CBD has been known to promote anandamide levels. It does so by inhibiting the enzyme that breaks down anandamide, maintaining higher anandamide levels and preventing bronchi obstruction.

CBD as a Preventative

Prevention is the best medicine, and studies show CBD has the potential to protect the lungs from asthmatic symptoms.

Cannabinoid receptors play the largest role in prevention. As the studies above concluded, activating these receptors has the potential to protect the lungs from becoming inflamed even when a trigger occurs. This would prevent patients from experiencing symptoms, allowing them to enjoy a normal life.

In addition, suppressing cytokine production and raising anandamide levels in the bronchial fluid could keep asthmatic symptoms at bay.

Asthma Patients Have Reason To Hope With CBD

Asthma is a serious illness and complicates the lives of its sufferers. With millions of patients in the US alone, and tens of millions more worldwide, it is important to offer hope by finding new therapies that provide relief for everyone.

CBD is providing new hope for those who cannot adequately manage their asthma with medication or do not wish to because of the potential side effects.

Despite limited research, CBD's therapeutic effects for the disease are promising, and previous studies prove

CBD is a safer treatment than pharmaceutical medication. Additionally, the CIITECH/Hebrew University of Jerusalem study should encourage patients that the cannabinoid's benefits for the disease may soon be solidified.

As further research is confirming, CBD is a promising therapy for asthma and will help many patients lead happier, healthier lives.

Preliminary research shows that CBD may help with or to minimize the inflammation that is experienced by asthma patients. Asthma is an atopic severe condition. That means it causes immediate allergic reactions. This chronic severe condition causes the airways to be inflamed more often leading to the restriction of airflow. It is characterized by difficulties in breathing, chest tightness, wheezing, and coughing. Inflammation and swelling makes airways of the patient prone to allergic reactions and more sensitive. Though asthma can be a minor health issue in some people, it can be a serious problem that affects the daily lives of others. Unfortunately, there is no conventional cure for asthma at the moment.

HOW CBD COULD POTENTIALLY RELIEVE ASTHMA

Although more research needs to be conducted to establish the effectiveness of CBD in improving the symptoms of asthma, early research indicates that CBD has showed promising results when used to relieve asthma. According to early research, the anti-inflammatory properties of CBD enable it to minimize inflammation among asthma patients.

Additionally, studies have shown that CBD reduces TH2 and TP cytokines levels. They also suggest that CBD might influence response in major mucus hyper-secretion stimuli. This is another prominent symptom that is experienced by asthma patients.

The findings of the recent studies are consistent with those of early studies. All indicate that CBD has anti-inflammatory and immunosuppressive properties. Some studies have also shown that CBD reduces asthma-related pain. This is very important considering the fact that severe pain that results from asthma attacks can be very uncomfortable, or even debilitating in some patients.

However, it should be noted that though there are no pain receptors within the lungs, asthma patients experience pain due to their inability to breathe. Interruption of normal airflow causes additional stress on the accessory muscles like scalene and sternocleidomastoid. CBD alleviates this pain by reducing muscle spasticity and pressure in the lungs.

USING CANNABIDIOL TO RELIEVE ASTHMA SYMPTOMS

Finally, it has been documented that CBD can be used as a potent therapeutic aid for asthma relief. When used in any method, CBD decreases airways resistance. However, it's important to use CBD with care. Ideally, you should make sure that the CBD that you use is isolated, and not mixed with THC. That's because THC is responsible for the high feeling that is associated with cannabis. CBD, on the other hand, does not cause this feeling.

www.ingramcontent.com/pod-product-compliance
Lightning Source LLC
Chambersburg PA
CBHW051413250726
48655CB00003B/1019